Intro

I believe every woman CAN squirt. Even though every woman is different, the basic anatomy is the same for most. Ergo, if one can, they all can. Just my opinion, and I share that opinion knowing that since I am a man, I may never truly know what I'm talking about 100% when it comes to the female body. I want to repeat. This is only my experience with the subject. I have lots of experience (about 35 years worth), but make no claim that I know everything. And, there are probably many women who have had experiences that differ from what I'm about to detail. This primer is the body of my experience.

Series Table Of Contents

Part 1: Intro
    Anthropology
    How Porn Got Us Into It

Part 2: Oh, The Pressure!
    Making Her Squirt
    Getting Comfy

Part 3: Anatomy & How To

Part 4: Arousal
    Orgasm vs Squirting

Part 5: It's Not Pee!!
    Some notes on the smell and taste

Part 6: Go Big Or Go Home
    Water Cannons, Fisting and Stretching

Anthropology

I think that many, many, many years ago, female ejaculation was probably the normal and natural way that a woman experienced sex. It was probably as normal and natural as a man ejaculating. There is probably a biological reason for it beyond just adding lubrication and keeping the vagina clean, which are the most common theories. Something like, it improves the odds of fertilization. Or, the unique blend of chemicals in female ejaculation perform a health function of some kind. That makes sense to me since the original purpose of sex is survival of the species.

We made it fun, thank goodness. Us and the dolphins (and maybe some of the monkeys) are the only creatures that do it for fun. That's according to those that study animal husbandry. I'm not sure I agree with that completely. Lions fuck something like 500 times a day. I have a difficult time believing it's all for baby lions. But, that's what they say. So, it makes sense that the original purpose had something to do with making more people.

A woman I talked to recently offered a theory that female ejaculation may be a remaining gift that had a purpose no longer needed. We have evolved the reason out of us. There are several parts of the human body that are no longer required for survival, like the appendix. Maybe squirting is another characteristic of the body that once provided some vital function, but now, does not.

She also proposed that squirting may have been involved in asexual reproduction. Many organisms reproduce asexually, although no mammals that I know of. But if we go back far enough in evolutionary history, her idea is very possible. All DNA boils down to a series of choices similar to "on" "off" switches. Scientists studying gene sequencing have found evidence that we still contain the genes for regrowing limbs and gills and other characteristics that have long ago been permanently switched "off". Could the anatomy (and reason) for squirting be from some point in prehuman history? I am very open to that possibility.

She also introduced the word epigenetics, which was a word from so far back in my education I had to refresh myself on the topic. LOL. But once I caught up, her idea got me thinking and theorizing on my own. Asexual reproduction produces carbon copy offspring since there is no outside variable of the second parent, or combination of the genetic contribution of grandparents, great-grandparents, etc. Epigenetics is the study of those variables, which wouldn't exist. Maybe squirting, which is influenced by environmental factors such as the mother's diet, could introduce the variable possibilities. Maybe. Without something to introduce those variables, evolution would never occur since all offspring would be identical. Those variables, at every stage, brought us from single cell organisms to where we are now. Could female ejaculation be a vital function at some stage? Possibly.

Just for grins, I did some research to see if I could find any other organisms where the females of the species ejaculates. As you can imagine, I didn't find much. But, what I DID find was volumes of information about multiple sea creatures that "eject" eggs (sometimes fertilized, other times not, sometimes fertilized asexually) from their bodies for gestation in some manner. Could that be the origin of female ejaculation? Possibly. I doubt we'll ever know for sure though.

Back to the current female humans. Thousands of years of human history where women were told it's not ladylike to enjoy sex, squirting, and even female orgasm, has been sort of "bred out" of the female sexual experience. We actually made it so that women have to LEARN how to orgasm and learn how to ejaculate. Books on the subject were considered pornographic. Many women went their entire lives and never had a single orgasm, and only had sex because it was their "wifely duty". Some may have had an orgasm or two over the years. Some may have experienced ejaculation (and were considered freaks, which was NOT a good thing in those days). It happened usually by happy accident when women masturbated. Rarely did it happen by design, when they had sex with their husbands.

Women have had to LEARN how to make it happen intentionally. Once they learn how, it blends back into their natural sexual behavior and becomes easier. But at first, instead of being able to just enjoy what is normal and natural, many women have to "learn" how. Where are the books and videos telling men how to orgasm and ejaculate? Exactly. Most men don't know how to bring a woman to orgasm, even if they learn the mechanics of what SHOULD make it happen. Orgasm is a cerebral event and women's brains work differently than men's brains. It is really only in the last 30-40 years that female orgasm (and ejaculation) has been reborn as a topic that is socially acceptable to talk about. Thank goodness!! Right?

How Porn Got Us Into It

Someone I talked to recently said, "There's no better way of taking the pulse of society in different countries than looking at their porn."

So now, add porn. Squirting has had a meteoric rise in adult entertainment. Let me digress for a moment. At one time, it WAS a lot of peeing. Porn was the first to learn that if you drink TONS of water and completely flush the bladder, the pee that comes out is completely clear and can mimic ejaculation. It's called water loading. When the scene calls for the big squirt, she simply pees. For greater effect, she "pushes" hard and fakes an orgasm. And wallah!! A whole new genre was born.

But you have to think. Porn didn't just make this up one day. There HAD to be some women who squirted naturally. Porn got wind of it and instead of trying to figure out how it works to recreate it naturally, they came up with the water loading trick. At first, squirting was such a freaky thing that no one even knew how to mimic it believably. Water loading was the best they could come up with.

There are several things you have to think about before we start comparing what we see in a video to real life. First, what woman can relax enough to squirt naturally her first time with a camera crew and a cast of people milling around? And second, it is nearly impossible to "perform" as we expect porn actresses to perform WHILE having a genuine orgasm. In the video, it's fairly easy to recognize (if you've ever been present when a woman has an orgasm), that she probably isn't having one. She is ACTING. She is a trained professional PERFORMING a sex act for your entertainment.

We want the squirt though, as the symbolic, visual evidence of the orgasm she is supposedly having (like the "money shot" with men). So, water loading continues for the ones who can't do it naturally on cue, with a room full of people, and make it look spectacular. Lucky for those who enjoy squirt porn, these days, it is mostly real squirting, due to a few women leading the education on the topic.

Once a few women who genuinely squirt by honest means came forward and began to openly discuss it to enlighten others, more and more women (and adult film actresses) learned how and now it is mostly true ejaculation. Many of these women have learned to UNsynchronize squirting and orgasm to be able to perform as expected. I'll come back to that. And, I'll come back to how you can tell when it's water loading and when it's natural. See the chapters on Anatomy and Orgasms.

You also have to remember that having an orgasm while holding a full bladder is a difficult trick in itself. Add to that, the nerves that go along with having an orgasm while performing all the other choreography of the scene IN FRONT OF A ROOM FULL OF PEOPLE, and you'll be able to figure out how real the orgasms mostly are. Not that it never happens; it does. It just doesn't happen the way it is portrayed. Remember, female adult film performers are human beings. They have all the same nervousness and hangups that everyone else does. Their profession usually helps them work through those and they are less of a hinderance to performing their jobs. BUT, they are still human beings.

Our porn shows something that often conflicts with real life experience. And instead of going with our personal experience with squirting, or taking the time to learn what's real, some people put two-and-two together for a sum of 5. You cannot draw any real world conclusions from what you see in a fantasy world. Keep your expectations between the video and real life realistic.

Oh, The Pressure!

I called an adult film actress I know who is known for her legendary squirting ability, and asked her about the pressure. YES!!! Even porn stars feel the pressure to perform. Yes, almost every female fan that has ever contacted her said, "My boyfriend/husband/lover/partner wants me to learn how. Please help me."

And so now, in real life, millions of women are feeling the pressure. Either they are comparing themselves to a friend who claims to squirt and claims how wonderful ti is, and she is trying to keep up with her peers. Or, her boyfriend/husband/lover/partner has seen it in a video and thinks he can MAKE her squirt or there's something wrong with HER if he can't. Or, her husband/boyfriend/lover/partner has confessed a fantasy about it and she wants to please him. Bless her heart.

Are women feeling pressure from their PARTNERS to squirt? Or do they put the pressure on themselves "to perform" and feel like they have failed when they don't? Basically, where does the pressure come from? I am betting that the overwhelm- ing answer to these questions is YES, from their partners, themselves, society, peers, everyone. Not only do women have to do everything listed, but NOW, they have to ejaculate like a geyser, too? Yup. But hey, no pressure.

It's a paradox for any woman who has never experienced it and is wanting to learn how. On one hand, they are told what an amazing thing it is. Most women who have experienced it report what a much more natural, fulfilling sexual experience it is to ejaculate. Most women who have learned how (or naturally were able to), say that now, they can't imagine NOT squirting. So, any woman who hears that is going to feel SOME pressure to "get there" and that they are missing out if they don't. And yes, to some degree, probably feel like they have failed every time they try and don't get there. They probably feel like they have let themselves and/or their partners down.

Add it to having cellulite, or less than perfect skin, or a body that doesn't fit some perfect image they think they SHOULD have, but don't, or any one of the millions of ways that women may not feel good enough. Add in the many women who seem to easily get there and are able to squirt WITHOUT having to read volumes of information and spend hours trying to learn "how". Sure, there's pressure.

Add to it the meteoric rise in squirting in EVERY form of adult entertainment. So, every time the husband/boyfriend/lover/ partner watches a video, the pressure is back and the feeling that she is somehow inadequate.

The paradox is that in order for them to get there, they need to NOT have the pressure. Of the women who are trying to learn, what is the ONE thing everyone says to help them? R-E-L-A-X. Really? "Drop an immense weight on me and then tell me to relax? Thanks. That's very helpful."

I don't know how many threads I've seen that begin with "I'm trying to learn how..." Every time I see those posts, I wonder "Why?" Have they seen something in porn and decided they want to learn how? Did their partner express a desire for the woman to learn? Maybe the idea came from a friend or peer who told her that she could squirt, or had learned to squirt and now she wants to keep up with her friend. I don't know. I'm curious to hear where the idea came from. Knowing that, might help us, who are trying to help her learn, be able to take that pressure off a little and help her relax. Maybe a little.

By the way, I am SOOOOOOOOOO glad to see some women post that they DON'T feel any pressure to squirt and that it isn't a big deal. The truth is, it's NOT a big deal if a woman doesn't. It's great for us men because we can say, "Cool! Look what I made her do!" It's more cool because most men have no earthly idea if a woman reached orgasm or not and their entire sexual self esteem is wrapped up in the goal instead of the journey and THEY feel like they failed, as a man, if they don't make their woman have a million orgasms every time they touch her. That certainly takes the pressure off, doesn't it ladies?

In my book, if a woman is healthy and happy and having fun, who needs the pressure? Every woman says it's a more satisfying orgasm. But, if a woman is very happy with the orgasms she is having, is adding the additional performance necessary? As her lover, it isn't my responsibility to MAKE her cross the line. Make her happy, yes. That's my job. But take it to the next level if she's already happy? I don't know.

Truthfully, ANY time pressure is applied to reaching a "goal", there will always be failure. This time, she only came once. Not good enough. This time, she only dribbled a little squirt. Not good enough. This time, it took her an hour of her lover barking at her for that one orgasm. Not good enough. Unless it is monumentally epic in scale, it will always be less than the goal. It's nice to focus on improvement and always wanting to do more or do better. That's ambition. Nothing wrong with that. But, pressure to achieve some unrealistic image of what should be will always result in the feeling of failure.

By the way, men, as we get older, we're not always going to be able to "perform" perfectly either. Oh go ahead, tell me it NEVER happens to you. I'll shine the S on your chest and bow down to you as my hero (while I call you a liar in my head). It DOES happen - to EVERY man - more so as we get older, but even healthy, young bucks. So, every time you put pressure on a woman to spray impressive fountains, remember karma. But hey, no pressure. It NEVER happens to you. Right?

That said, squirting is cool. Personally, I love it. I wish every woman squirted like a geyser every time I touched her. If nothing else, just for my own ego. Like every man, I want to feel like a god in the bedroom. Luckily, I have learned that what's truly important is how she feels when we're laying there in the afterglow. Is she happy? REALLY happy? No matter what happened? If she is, I'm happy too. I've been with a lot of women when things didn't go perfect and one of us, or even both of us, didn't feed any legends with our performance. It happens. Less than legendary is still awesome as long as everyone enjoyed what happened. THAT is what's important. As long as people are having fun and enjoying the time they're spending together, no one failed.

MY suggestion - and I have said this before in comments and posts - is approach things as an exploration and see what happens. No pressure to perform or achieve ANYTHING, except a better understanding of her body. Use the fingers to just learn the "landscape" and what feels good. Turn the cell phone off. Put some nice music on. Get a bottle of wine (and maybe even something to snack on because you'll want to be there a while). Talk and laugh. Lots of laughing. Lots of talking. Take. Your. Time. Just explore. The goal is NOT to squirt. Or even have an orgasm, not even one. Just learn. Enjoy the journey.

Because, the ONE thing that will guarantee to reduce the pressure, is intimacy and comfort. Taking the time to learn her body (or your own body if you're doing this sans partner), without any expectation of a performance, will build intimacy. Trust and comfort level does more to help her relax than anything else - especially telling her over and over and over to relax.

Making Her Squirt

Question: "How can I MAKE my girlfriend/wife/sub squirt?"

Question: "How can I MAKE my girlfriend/wife/sub let go and squirt?"

Question: "How can I MAKE my girlfriend/wife/sub relax enough to squirt?"

Since posting the first article on the topic, I have received this question no lees than a dozen times a day. It is usually accompanied by exhausting stories about how they have tried to FORCE their female partner to ejaculate like they see in porn and it just hasn't happened as expected.

In many cases, it is a lover who genuinely doesn't understand how it works and is sincerely looking for help. In many cases though, it is a wannabe Dom who thinks by demanding it, it will happen magically. Or, his ego is so huge that he thinks if he learns some special mechanics of the task, he will become a sex god that makes the magic happen. Some of these stories include how they commanded her to, "OPEN YOUR HOLE!" And, "DO IT NOW!" And for some reason, she just wouldn't. "Why the fuck not? What's wrong with HER?"

Let me say that AFTER a woman has some experience with ejaculation, barking orders at her as part of your D/s play is fine and you're likely to get the results you want. But, starting out, and the first time, that is all extremely counter productive. With experience, many women learn to adapt their abilities to all kinds of play. Women squirt when they are spanked. Women squirt when they have anal sex. Actually, LOTS of women squirt when they have anal sex. Women squirt from breast and/or nipple stimulation. Women squirt just about any time they have an orgasm, from whatever type of stimulation that brings them the orgasm. My favorite are the women who orgasm and squirt when giving head. And some, who have mastered psycholagny, can orgasm and squirt just by thinking about it.

Starting out though, let it suffice to say that it has to begin with baby steps. Progress should be measured humbly and HER process to get there has to be respected. If you try to force something, it usually breaks. In this case, the more force you apply, the more difficult it will be for her to let go. The more pressure she feels, the less she will be able to relax. If she can't relax, it won't happen.

That said, there ARE some women who learn to squirt from forced orgasms. This is a MUCH smaller number of women. There are also some guys who have been successful with this technique just enough that they honestly believe this is how it works. This would greatly be the exception to the rule. Once a woman has experience with squirting, forced orgasms work as well as other kinds of orgasms. Starting out, the more successful technique is to provide an environment where she can fully relax. mentally as well as physically.

It isn't a matter of "convincing her" to let go. You have to give her an environment that allows her to relax and feel comfortable, AND be okay with whatever happens naturally. Pushing is counter productive. The more you push, the more pressure you put on her. The more you tell her that it's okay to let go, the more pressure you put on her. It actually works the opposite, by making it very NOT okay to let go.

Pressure also translates into pressure-to-perform. It's like telling a man to hurry up and get a hardon. "DO IT NOW!!" Enough of that and you'll actually start to have a little ED. Same effect. Statements like, "OPEN YOUR HOLE!" can be playful in the right relationship dynamic. But, if you're trying to get your girlfriend to relax, probably a little crude and demanding. Results: NOT relaxed enough to open her hole.

Also remember that many women are extremely self conscious about squirting. Especially if it's new to her. Many women are self conscious about just letting you SEE their girl parts, let alone relaxed enough with it to completely let go with an audience. Blame society. The world puts unbelievable, unfair pressure on women to be perfect and ladylike. Squirting (letting go completely and making a mess) probably doesn't seem very ladylike and probably doesn't fit that social model.

Compound that with a lack of information, or poor information. There is a staggering amount of information on the internet that says that female ejaculation is urine. IT IS NOT URINE!! Yet, if you Google it, you'll find as much information that says that it is as information that says that it is not. So, see this from her side. You say, "Relax honey and let go." She hears, "Venture into unknown territory, get VERY uncomfortable with an audience, and PEE all over the bed." Personally, in her shoes, I would be very NOT convinced to let go.

Experienced squirters have learned that squirting is as empowering for her as it can get. But starting out, it's just the opposite. YOU have to give her that. But, you do that, by not really doing anything except being a comfortable man to explore that self-empowerment with. Chances are very good, if this is a relationship that you've been in for a while, that she WANTS to please you. She WANTS to give you what you want. If she's been around for a while, she's already decided you're PROBABLY okay to let go with. If you continue being that guy, eventually she'll get there. If you continue putting pressure on her, she never will. You have to be patient and let her get there on her own.

This will all sound like social media platitudes, but they all apply. Relax and enjoy the moment, no matter how it happens and whatever happens. Enjoy HER, whether she squirts or not. Focus on being the kind of man she WANTS to squirt for, not the man that is putting pressure on her, which makes her feel like a failure when she doesn't perform as YOU want. Most of all, just enjoy the journey, with or without squirting. The more you make it about a goal, the less likely you are to achieve it.

Getting Comfy

Relaxing is tricky. No one can really even help you very much because it's YOUR comfort that you have to figure out. Usually, with experience, that comfort comes easier. Many women that I've talked to started with masturbation. They get the hang of it and then introduce a partner. Alone gives you the opportunity to work on what makes you most comfortable AND what doesn't. Then, when you include a partner, you have some of those things figured out. Being with a partner can greatly inhibit whatever works when you're alone. Different things work for different women. So, I believe it's not some special sexual technique, but what happens in the brain that triggers it.

Trust your instincts. If it makes you uneasy, eliminate it, even if it seems stupid. For example, I had a girlfriend that couldn't squirt with the ceiling fan on, with me or by herself. She could have an orgasm, but not ejaculate. The ceiling fan distracted her and prevented her from fully letting go. Another one, the pillows had to be arranged a certain way. I just talked to someone recently that told me when she first started squirting, she could ONLY squirt in the kitchen because there was a tile floor and she could easily clean up the mess. In the kitchen, she felt free and could squirt "like a fire hydrant" from just about any kind of stimulation.

With experience, distractions and the stuff in your head that keeps you from relaxing WILL get better. I think everyone with more experience will confirm that. But in the beginning, you might have to work on removing distractions first (mental and environmental). There's plenty of nice people in the squirting groups to talk to that can share their experience. But, you're the only one in your head. Ultimately, you'll need to identify whatever it is that bothers you and address it.

It's true, some techniques seem to work better than others for the majority, starting out. But that doesn't really explain why the same techniques don't work on ALL women, all the time since anatomically, most women (generally speaking) are a lot alike. And, if it was a universal methodology, following that methodology would make all men sexual gods just by learning steps from a book.

I also believe it has to do with a woman's experience. The more experienced a woman is with squirting, the wider the range of activities that can trigger it. My theory, and I want to emphasize that it's just my theory, is that the brain makes an association between the physical stimulation and the mental process that occurs. More experience, the more familiarity there is with that process and the ability to apply that process to an expanded arena of stimulation. Basically, the more you do it, the more you learn about it and the better you get at doing it, and the better you get at recreating the results applied to a wider range of stimuli. Just my theory based on experience. See the chapter on Orgasms.

I think a lot of it happens on a subconscious level. That mental association with the things that impair it or trigger it. Which is why being able to relax and let go is the most common advice everyone shares. I think when a woman relaxes, it allows that subconscious process to occur more easily. No matter the comfort with a partner, almost every woman that I've talked to was less relaxed (to some degree) with a partner than they are when alone. At first, you have to stop worrying about pleasing your partner, and stop worrying, "Am I doing this right?" For some women, this means to completely switch gears. You have to stop worrying about how your partner will react. You have to stop worrying about the mess, and anything else you're worrying about. Yes, I know, telling you to stop worrying is the surest guarantee that you're not going to stop worrying. But, the paradox is what it is.

As a friend said, "Sometimes, it's difficult to get into the relaxed place you need to be when you're doing the work." And so, for some women, working with a partner actually makes it EASIER to get there. They're able to relax and just enjoy the stimulation provided by their partner and let go. You might have to experiment both ways to find your threshold for getting there. Once there, you'll likely find squirting to be very natural and easy. And once there, being alone or with a partner will deliver the same results.

Question: "My boyfriend wants me to squirt and tells me it's okay if it's pee. I can't get past the pee thing to let go and squirt."

Answer: Ask yourself what it is that bothers you about it. It is probably a list of things. Tackle each one by itself. See if you can resolve it. Maybe use puppy pads to take care of the mess. Maybe rethink the concept in some way. Things like that. But make a list and address each item one at a time. Communicate with your partner too. Instead of him just telling you it's great, have him help you break it down and work through it. one piece at a time.

The thinking that it's urine is often the most difficult hurdle to overcome. It isn't urine. Sadly, there is as much information on the internet that says that it is, as there is saying that it isn't. See Chapter 5 for on that.

Learning to squirt is like getting to the top of a hill. The pressure makes it like a blind, confusing, stressful mad dash. But once you get to the top of that hill, everything becomes easy. From the summit, you can see all the paths up and down the hill and can choose the ones that work best. Kinda like being able to look down from the top of that hill and see an amazing playground with a million options to play with. BUT, you have to get to the top of that hill the first time. And paradoxically, you get there not with a mad dash, but with a very comfortable, relaxing stroll.

Anatomy & How To

The g-spot is kinda behind the clit on the inside. Visualize a line extending from the clit running up and inside. There's the g-spot. If you lay on your back and insert a finger, feel along the "top" of the vaginal canal and you'll feel several spongy ridges. That's the urethral sponge. Then around the top of that urethral sponge (generally), you will probably feel something like a "dip". There's the g-spot. A g-spot orgasm may not necessarily be from direct stimulation of that spot, but from stimulation of that spongy area, which indirectly stimulates the g-spot. It's very similar to how stimulating your clitoral hood and the area AROUND your clit gets you off but direct stimulation on the clit is often too intense. Same kinda thing.

Squirting is most commonly from vigorous stimulation of that spongy area, not necessarily the g-spot. Using your middle two fingers, make a "come hither" motion from that dip, along the ridges. Many references show people doing this with the index and middle finger. That's fine, but...

1) The fingers folded that way causes tension on the muscles in the hand and forearm and the hand and arm will get tired much, much sooner;

2) If a woman is masturbating and exploring her own body, to use those two fingers involves cranking your wrist in a very unnatural position;

3) Using those two fingers (by a partner) tends to cause the hand to naturally "rotate" which changes the contact to the spongy area (urethral sponge) and reduces the effectiveness of the stimulation;

4) The hand turned can make contact with the outer labia, inner labia and vaginal opening in a way that can be more distracting than pleasurable but using the middle and ring finger leaves the index and pinky finger up and out of the way; and

5) Using the middle and ring finger allows for a variety of stimulation techniques, but the other way - even when properly positioned - really only allows for the one stimulation technique.

Anyway, I digress. Apply FIRM pressure with the fingers as you do that "come hither" motion. Oh, for the love of God, TRIM YOUR NAILS THOROUGHLY before you EVER stick your fingers inside another person's body!!! Jus' sayin'. With practice, the person doing the stimulating can learn to alternate circular motions and rubbing motions along with the come hither to bridge between moments of intense stimulation. That's important for beginners because the sensations can be incredibly intense.

Build, rest, repeat. Intense stimulation for a while, then gentle stimulation, then intense, etc. It is very unlikely to have an orgasm from the intense stimulation in a way that she isn't familiar with. Remember, sex for most women is as much a mental event as it is a physical one. There will be A LOT going on in her brain while this is taking place. That mental processing is REQUIRED for her to learn how. Guys, that's just the way women work. Trying to force the process actually guarantees it won't happen. So, stimulate, relax, stimulate and relax. And if nothing happens, don't sweat it. Give it a rest and try again another time. With some experience, the doors are wide open to how to do things. But at first, remember that this is a new experience that she must MENTALLY process for it to be successful. Pressure and forcing her is a strategy for it to be UNsuccessful.

If you are first learning to squirt, stimulation of your urethral sponge may cause the sensation that you need to pee. This can be a little confusing for the inexperienced. First, you're told to drink LOTS of water. So, actually needing to pee is always a possibility. Second, because you aren't familiar with the sensation of ejaculation, your brain identifies the sensations with something you already know: peeing. Urinating may feel like the same thing until you learn the difference.

The urethral sponge does two things. By contracting, like any other muscle, it squeezes the urethra and holds urine in. AND, also by contacting, it pushes ejaculate out. The brain only knows about holding in urine. So, when the sponge is stimulated, the brain thinks it is holding in urine, which means, you need to pee. With practice, you can learn the difference between the sensations and your brain will identify them easier.

Needing to pee can be distracting, thus keeping you from letting go. And, needing to pee can also create anxiety about making a mess, which also keeps you from relaxing and letting go. Get around this by making sure you completely empty your bladder before you engage in some squirting practice. And, use some puppy pads. That way, even if you do pee, there's no mess that can't be managed. Pee washes out easily from towels, sheets, comforters, etc. The important thing is that you MUST relax to let go, and needing to pee - whether that's really the case or just the brain identifying the same sensation - can be a huge deterrent.

Squirting and ejaculation are the same thing. Squirt is not urine. It is the same fluid that your vagina uses for lubrication. See the chapter on this. Urine exits the body from the bladder via the urethra. Ejaculation exits the body from the urethral sponge via the paraurethra, also well know as the Skeen's Glands or Skene's Glands.

Bartholin's Glands might help the vagina lubricate, but generally not much. Maybe earlier in human history. they were more functional for that. Now, their purpose has evolved and they really don't do much of anything anymore, except provide the most modest amount of lubrication to the vaginal opening. The paraurethral ducts provide a little more, but even though they are the exit door for all that squirt, the majority of vaginal lubrication seeps through the tissue of the vaginal walls (just inside the opening) when they become filled with blood from stimulation.

Let me take this moment to introduce a radical idea. Ladies, and I am speaking especially to the ones who have given birth, you know how you sometimes leak a little pee when you sneeze or cough? Kegels will help with that. But, this isn't about Kegels. My idea is that maybe it isn't pee. My idea is that maybe it is ejaculate.

Follow my train my thought. When you sneeze or cough, every muscle in your core contracts. That would include the urethral sponge. The urethral sponge contracts to hold pee in. It also contracts to squirt. What squirts is the vagina's natural lubrication, which collects in the urethral sponge. You don't necessarily have to be aroused for the body to produce that fluid. When the urethral sponge contracts, it sends that fluid out through the paraurethra. Is it possible that what you're leaking is natural vaginal fluid, not pee? I think sometimes it could be. Just an idea.

Squirting and orgasm are two separate events. For many, the two things synchronize and become one. But, that's actually a mental process, not a biological one. It is quite possible to squirt without orgasm just as you can orgasm without squirting, and starting out, many women do. What makes the two seem like part of the same event is that the motion for one can cause the other, and may cause both at the same time. It may happen that way for you as you learn how, but it may also just be one or the other. Many women say that they ejaculate just before or just after they peak at orgasm.

Even though the mechanics above are commonly what works, and every woman is GENERALLY similar (anatomically speaking), every woman is different, physically, emotionally and mentally. Your brain is as much to credit with success as any special skills your lover may have. Your brain can also be the greatest hinderance. Starting out, you MUST be relaxed and comfortable and be able to completely let go without reservation. If your brain isn't in the right spot, all the skills and know-how in the world won't work. But once you're in the right place, almost anything will work.

All of this said, the best advice anyone can give someone wanting to learn to squirt is: 1) RELAX. No pressure to perform or achieve anything. And 2) EXPLORE your body with curiosity and a sense of adventure. No pressure to orgasm or squirt, just patiently learn and discover.

I believe most people discover what "works" for them by happy accident, not necessarily information or practicing some special technique. The more pressure someone applies to performance, the less likely someone is to perform. A woman's body is an amazing playground and the more exploration that is done, the more that will be learned. The more that is learned, the more pleasure it is possible to experience. Even if you discover some things don't do anything for you, you'll find all kinds of new things that will be amazing. Most of all, learning is fun for both people and everything you learn will compound with things you learn next time. Have fun!! That's what it's all about.

Arousal

Orgasm is what the brain does. Ejaculation is what the body does. The body squirts. The brain squirts oxytocin and serotonin into the system making you happy, giving you the feeling of euphoria. All of that begins with arousal, which takes place in, you guessed it, the brain. And by the brain, I mean, the ENTIRE brain. It seems that because arousal is so completely individualized, it could literally be any combination of brain cells coming to life when we are exposed to things that turn us on.

The brain's reward system, mostly in the cortico-basal ganglia-thalamo-cortical loop, perks up after a quick cognitive process. It starts with an appraisal of what we are presented with, a categorization of the stimulus as sexual, followed by a determination of what the proper response should be. From there, we usually make a decision to pursue or not pursue the stimulus to achieve the reward. For most people, that process would continue towards sexual activity with the eventual goal of orgasm. We also have procreative results that may or may not include an orgasm. And, sometimes we engage in the process for intimacy, also with or without an orgasm.

Most people think that men are quick to get aroused and women are much slower to become aroused. This is not true!! It is about equal in the process of becoming aroused. It takes different things to do it. But the speed and intensity are about the same. Of course, it is all dependent of what is appraised and categorized as being sexually interesting. This and that, and virtually every single thing in the world turns SOMEONE on. And, turns someone off. Depending on what it is that turns you on - what your brain decides is sexually interesting - that decides your individualized spectrum for arousal.

And, different things arouse different people for different reasons. Seeing a woman's breasts is a perfect example. You can be a completely straight woman, but women's breasts still fire up the arousal process. They do so for an entirely different reason than they do for straight men, but they still tap arousal on the shoulder. Even men who are completely gay also have an arousal response to women's breasts. Also for different reasons. These varied responses to the same stimuli, will light up a completely unique combination of neurons in the brain because they are appraised and evaluated so uniquely to the individual.

If you asked all 7-1/2 billion people on the planet what turns them on, you'd get 7-1/2 billion different answers. And then if you ask them an hour later, you might get 7-1/2 billion completely different answers. Sometimes, arousal is situational. Sometimes, it can have environmental influences such as where a person is or who they are with. Sometimes, it has to do with what happened right before you asked them. Sometimes it is opportunistic. It literally can be ANYTHING, ANY TIME, ANYWHERE.

Am I the only one who thinks it is very strange that, with all this potential for men and women to get turned on, that most people, most of the time, are having sex the same ol' way? Oh sure, many people have a wide range of kinks and fetishes and behavior to go along with their VERY individual turn ons.

Almost everyone has SOMETHING weird that turns them on in some way. We ALL do. We ALL have certain needs and desires and must-haves for the arousal response to carry us beyond the initial appraisal and categorization process. That criteria is incredibly unique to each person. So, why is most of our sex so NOT unique?

Let me throw one more oddity into the mix. The default setting for all of us begins exactly the same. It actually has nothing to do with sex. What we want is intimacy. We want to love someone and be loved by someone. That's it. Regardless of the individualization that takes place as we experience the world, we all start in the same place. And later, as we develop our unique set of needs and wants and must haves, no matter how strange they might seem, we can still reduce it down to how those activities satisfy our need for love.

Like six degrees to Kevin Bacon, and who DOESN'T love Kevin Bacon, all our kinks and fetishes and weirdness, no matter how vanilla or UNvanilla, can be traced back to that very essential origin. From there, life shows us a bunch of stuff and our brains make associations with that stuff. Some of it, we categorize as sexual and it gets added to our arousal process.

And if you're wondering how all that figures in with gay and straight people, it actually doesn't. Starting out, the default setting that just wants love, is about as pansexual as it gets. Long before we decide or recognize a primary attraction to one or the other, our little hearts and brains don't really care. Yes, some people are naturally mostly attracted to women and some are mostly attracted to men. But, it's kinda like the boobs. That pansexuality is still in there. We're still looking for the love from whatever source presents albeit for very personal reasons and criteria. Remove the labels, social conditioning, cultural standards, expectations and peer pressure, what turns us on is still quite open minded.

Our brain makes a connection to something that triggers the arousal response. That connection is based on experiences and thoughts. You might see boobs and get turned on. Something at some point has connected those two things, for example. That connection can be made to almost anything, though. I worked with a couple a while back. He was an auto mechanic and would kiss his wife passionately when he came home from work, usually before he showered. She developed a VERY intense arousal connection to the smell of the gunk that mechanics get all over them. That was great until the husband got promoted to manager and wasn't working on the cars anymore.

Sounds, smells, tastes are like brain-porn because they remind us of emotional experiences. Our emotions - deny them or not - control our arousal connections. Boobs make you feel at ease (for example) and that "at ease" feeling is really what triggers the arousal, not actually the sight of boobs. The smell of fresh baked apple pie might do the same thing. Or the sound of a car pulling up in the driveway. A lot of things that we would never consider sexual, all contribute to our arousal connections. Also, without a lot of those non sexual arousal connections, we might never get turned on even when we see boobs, because the very non sexual cues comfort us in the ways needed for us to connect with the sexual cues. Kinda like, settling distractions that block us from making the arousal connections.

Orgasm vs Squirting

Orgasm is the result of an association between the brain and body. Provide a known type of stimulation and the brain is pre-programmed to respond with an orgasm. It begins with a "default setting" for most people. A little of the ol' in 'n' out and wallah! But individually, we reprogram all the time. We all have hangups that interfere with the default setting. We all have fetishes and interests and turn ons that add to the default setting. For most people, especially women, the default setting doesn't work very well the way most men are "defaulting" it. They need some additional stimulation, or a different kind of stimulation to get them there.

All of that individualized programming is learned, as are all the things that interfere with people reaching orgasm. At some point, through some kind of life experience, THIS works and our brains remember it, and incorporates it into the equation. As we go through life, what works can change dramatically. As our range of life experiences change and as our bodies change, our "default setting" can proportionally change.

Orgasm occurs when the brain has associated something that will cause an orgasm. However, it is very common to have an orgasm from things that you wouldn't think should cause one. Holding hands or kissing or massaging her feet as common examples. I taught a woman to orgasm when her husband brushed her hair. My ex, and many other women, have developed the ability to orgasm and squirt on command without being touched, using auralism and/or visualization techniques. There's also psycholagny, one of my favorites.

Naturally, your brain makes the connection that brushing your hair should elicit an orgasm. Of course. Or brushing your teeth. Right? Okay. That is a little unusual, but that's kinda how it works. Cause and effect. Naturally, the brain makes the association with genital stimulation. THAT is the default setting. There are just as many nerves in your fingertips. Or your mouth. Why doesn't brushing our teeth cause an orgasm? Or simply holding the toothbrush? Hahaha. I just got a visual of a fetish where people get off on stroking the bristles of a toothbrush with their fingertips. Nevermind.

In women, arousal and orgasm is often triggered by emotional and mental stimulation as much as anything physical. Some men too, but women are so much better at this than men. The arousal response begins long before anything physical happens. And because of this, women can enjoy a much wider range of stimulation to bring them to orgasm. Literally, it is possible to orgasm from anything. I haven't met a woman yet who would orgasm from doing my laundry. I never say never though.

Psycholagny is the ability to reach or achieve orgasm without any physical stimulation of the genitalia, usually achieved through mental stimulation or fantasy alone. This is actually a lot easier than it might seem. It CAN be achieved by men as well as women, but I've seen overwhelmingly more success with women. My opinion is that we should ALL be able to achieve this easily, since orgasm is, after all, a mental process, not a physical one.

The process begins with arousal and ends with orgasm. This part is all cerebral and doesn't require any physical stimulation at all. With practice, it is possible to orgasm from literally anything. Laundry? (he jokes) Sure. Or walking on the treadmill. Or anything other chore you don't like. It's actually quite possible. Some foods and smells and sounds can give us pleasurable sensations because we have nice memories ASSOCIATED with them. Applying this process to anything takes practice, but with that practice, the possibilities are endless.

Separately, we have ejaculation. In men AND women, it is the physical response to stimulation. It works just like the orgasm response. Orgasm takes place in the brain and ejaculation takes place with the body. In men, generally, it works by default setting. For women, there may have been a default setting at some point in human history. I suspect there was. But now, it is a matter of re-associating the stimulus to the response.

You have to teach your brain that ejaculation is normal and natural. It IS, but your brain doesn't remember that. The most common way is to stroke the g-spot, or more accurately, the urethral sponge.

Once you learn to make it happen intentionally, it'll work just like with orgasms. You can apply this response process to virtually ANY stimuli. As you are learning and practicing, pay close attention to every sensation of the process from arousal to orgasm. Then practice application to other types of stimulation. That sounds crazy complicated and difficult. Try it. You'll learn that it's actually easier than it sounds.

When I said earlier that women can ejaculate from giving a blowjob, or with breast/nipple stimulation, or just by thought alone, this is actually more common than it sounds. Brushing your hair. Brushing your teeth. Virtually anything. This is why I'm optimistic about the laundry thing. I've treated quite a few anorgasmic women with helping them learn to "think" themselves to orgasm. By practicing application of this process, you create new, or even unconventional, associations as pathways to orgasm and/or ejaculation.

Since orgasm and ejaculation are the brain's associated response to a stimulus that it has associated with the two events, there is usually a close synchronization of the two. For almost all men, they reach orgasm just before they ejaculate. The timing is so close that it seems to be perfectly synchronized. This timing is generally believed to be for procreation. As the man is reaching his peak or orgasm, he is likely to leave his penis right where it is, insuring the most little swimmers will venture from his body into the woman's body.

For women, ejaculation can be just before or just after orgasm. It's still close enough that it seems to be well synchronized, even though it usually isn't exact. Most women have told me that the orgasm when they ejaculate is a "more satisfying" or "more complete" orgasm. It is like any other orgasm before was holding back a little. And even with some experience and they learn to control their squirting, many times they don't because the orgasm is less satisfying when they do.

Men don't need to be more turned on, am I right? We'd never get out of bed. But because you are infinitely better than men at the cerebral process from arousal to orgasm, women have infinite potential for application. It doesn't end with being able to squirt. It is just beginning. I am so jealous!! Talk about empowerment!!

And if you learn to orgasm and squirt just by thinking about it and/or from a wide range of stimulation, this makes you a VERY fun girl. Of course, if you find yourself squirting uncontrollably in line at the DMV, you might need to reel things back in a bit. Men think about sports to slow down ejaculating. You might need to try that, or consider memorizing the digits of Pi or thinking of solutions to a Rubik's Cube

It is possible to learn to improve the synchronization with practice. There is also nothing wrong with leaving it right where it is. Many women can ejaculate without any sign of an orgasm. And of course, most women have experienced orgasms without any sign of ejaculation. Basically, the brain associates one thing with the other. "It I experience THIS, I'm supposed to do THIS." Your brain can associate anything with anything else. Or, might NOT link two things. If, for whatever reason, your brain doesn't associate ejaculation and orgasm exactly together, then it won't happen together. Whatever your brain associates will act as a trigger for the event/activity. Your brain can associate ANYTHING as causing or NOT causing orgasm or ejaculation.

Starting out, just get there. Once you get there, with practice, you can learn to use it and control it like a super power.

It's Not Pee!!

One of the biggest hangups with women (and their lovers) when they first start exploring ejaculation is whether or not it's pee. There is as much INaccurate information about this online as there is accurate information. And sadly, even some of the bad information is coming from medical professionals. Sadly-er is the number of people who stop their research with one poorly researched, inaccurate article and draw a conclusion that it's urine without going any further, and then populate that information throughout the interweb wherever they go. Sadly-est is the number of people who do no research of any kind and still draw a conclusion based on the bad information. Most sadly-er of all is that female ejaculation isn't the only subject this is true with. Sigh.

There is research that concludes that female ejaculation is urine. That research was NOT performed in The scientific method. Meaning, they approached the research with a conclusion already in mind and set out to prove it by designing the research to only reach that conclusion. Those that have performed reputable scientific research have concluded that it is NOT urine. Female ejaculation does not exit the body from the urethra, which is the ONLY way urine comes out. It exits from the paraurethra, or also called Skene's glands or Skeens glands. The composition of female ejaculate is almost exactly the same as the natural lubrication of the vagina.

Ejaculation is not urine. I repeat. It is not urine. It is not urine. It is not urine. Anyone who thinks it is should be excommunicated until they get their head out of their ass. Because female ejaculation exits the body NEAR the urethra (via the paraurethral ducts or lacunae), there might possibly be trace amounts of urine, but no more so than the amount of urine that is in a man's ejaculate. In fact, probably less because male ejaculate come out of the same exit as urine. Female ejaculate does not.

The composition of female ejaculate is mostly water, just as her natural lubrication is. But, the fluid also commonly contains urea, creatinine, prostatic acid phosphatase (PAP), prostate specific antigen (PSA), pyridine, squalene, acetic acid, lactic acid, glycol, ketone, and aldehyde, glucose and fructose in varying amounts (usually varied by a woman's diet). Some of the same chemicals CAN BE present in urine and vice versa.

And yes, sometimes there might be a little bit of pee. Back to some anatomy. One of the primary functions of the urethral sponge is to help with incontinence. So, "pushing" out the ejaculate and urinating are similar functions, biologically speaking. Ejaculation is kind of an involuntary act by the body and when that sponge starts working to "push", any urine in the bladder can also be pushed out. But, these are still two separate things. The ejaculate is one fluid. Urine is another. This is where much of the confusion in the medical community occurs. Examination of a puddle underneath the woman who just squirted a gallon or so, can give very mixed results.

I have several pieces of advice for this fact. First, if you're squeamish about bodily fluids (pee including), you may want to avoid sex altogether. Pee won't hurt you. Society tells us it's unacceptable to get it on you or touch it, but unless the person has some kind of medical issue, urine is perfectly safe. There are actually lots of people who drink it and claim all kinds of health benefits. "Golden showers" and other descriptors of urine play are common fetishes. Although I'm sure someone somewhere has suffered a medical issue as a result, I have yet to hear of such a situation. The biggest problem with pee is what happens in our brains because of the societal stigma, not because of any biological issue.

If you're still concerned with whether or not it's pee and unsettled by a little of it possibly getting on you, go play with girls who don't squirt. Squirt, and urine, washes out of everything. Have towels, or a tarp, handy. And just my opinion, if other people's bodily fluids freak you out, stick to masturbation.

Once a woman has some experience with squirting, and practices, she can usually tell the difference between urinating and squirting and can learn to control each. It helps immensely if she does plenty of Kegels.

I recently spoke to a woman who can PROVE 100% that squirting is not urine. She is into sounding. I asked her if she had ever squirted with a sound inside her. She said she has. BUT, you have to firmly hold the sound in to keep it from shooting across the room like a projectile and putting someone's eye out. Word of caution to anyone trying this: Safety first!!

Since urine ONLY exits the body from the urethra, a sound plugging the urethra means that it can't possibly be urine (at least in her case). If you still believe that female ejaculation is urine, try a urethral plug or sound. Prove me wrong (as well as almost any woman who squirts). Since originally posting about this, several women have talked to me about squirting with a sound in and have the same story to share.

Some others have told me about squirting with a catheter fully inserted. Once again, they were able to spray an impressive geyser while any urine went into the catheter. I've seen that video and I'm convinced.

Similar to orgasm denial or bathroom denial, it is possible to learn to squirt with an overwhelming need to urinate WITHOUT losing a drop of urine. I've talked to two women who have learned to do this. It took considerable practice. But eventually, they managed to do it. That's another way to know that ejaculation and urination are different things.

One of the mysteries that has yet to be discovered is where all that fluid comes from. If you believe that ejaculation is urine, how do you explain the volume when it exceeds the capacity of the bladder? The average female bladder holds a max of 600 ml, or about 2-/12 cups. In porn, in conversation, AND IN PERSON, I have witnessed a volume of ejaculation that was way more than that.

I have an ex that filled a bathtub 1/2" deep in a single session. There is no way that all came out of her bladder!! Same woman could spray like a geyser - just like in porn. She could hit the ceiling when she was in piledriver position and it would drip down on us for a while. She could hit the wall about 10' away at head height. It would drip down and soak the carpet. In both of those cases, the volume exceeded the max bladder capacity of 2-1/2 cups.

My ex wife didn't squirt from ANY kind of vaginal stimulation no matter what we tried. But when she was penetrated anally, she would squirt buckets. Each time, the volume was unbelievable. I can only estimate, but again, it exceeded the 2-1/2 cups.

I have a friend that squirted so much during a fisting session in my kitchen, that we had to take a break and mop the floor to keep everyone safe. Again, WAY more than the 2-1/2 cups. My kitchen tile floor, an area about 5' x 10', was covered!! It ran under my refrigerator and stove, and for days after, I was still mopping it up.

An adult film performer I am friends with brags that she can squirt a gallon a day. Her partner, another prolific squirter, claims they have tested that theory and proven it to be correct. Together, they are VERY learned in the genre of squirting and pee. They are convinced it is not urine. They also bring up the volume and say their bladders simply cannot hold that much at a time.

I challenged them to duplicate their tests using pee. Drink a lot of water and continue drinking as much water as they could hold and see if they could PEE as much as they squirt. They could not. This surprised them, so they tried again several times. Each time, testing urine and ejaculation on separate days, and each time, they could squirt much more than they could pee.

Another point they made was that having sex with a full bladder is not comfortable. And, to orgasm with a full bladder is nearly impossible. If the fluid that shoots out of a woman's body is urine and it is coming from her bladder, that makes the thousands of testimonies of women who say squirting accompanies an orgasm, a lie. C'mon. Thousands of women, independently, all telling the exact same lie to many, many sources? I have a hard time believing that.

The logic that ejaculation is urine would suggest that women pee when they orgasm. I don't know of any women who do, except those who also pee a little when they sneeze. LOL. It happens. Do your Kegels and it'll be all right.

The most believable theory (to me, and I have stated this throughout many of my posts) is that female ejaculate is the same fluid as a woman's natural lubrication. If you've ever had a marathon session with a woman, where she just stayed wet for an hour or so, imagine the volume of that fluid. Once again, an amount that I believe exceeds the 2-1/2 cups of the bladder. Where does that fluid come from? What part of her body produces or holds that fluid?

We know THAT fluid builds in the vaginal tissue and secretes through the porous tissue into the vaginal opening. Everybody has a theory, but no one truly seems to know for sure where that fluid originates, how it's stored and how the tissue regulates or disperses the fluid. Not being able to confirm anything with medical certainty opens the door for the people who theorize that it must be filling in the bladder, and thus, it must be urine.

The theory I subscribe to is that the fluid collects in the urethral sponge and when the sponge is stimulated, it contracts, ejecting the fluid out via the Skene's Glands. My theory is based on two facts. The first being the composition of the fluid is the same as the natural lubricating fluid of the vagina. And the second is that the fluid exits the body through the paraurethra (Skene's Glands) and they are not attached to the bladder or urethra. They are attached to the urethral sponge.

All I can do is shrug. I'm well versed in female anatomy and I have a long list of very educated sources. No one seems to have a theory that everyone can agree to as being plausible. The only thing we agree on is that it isn't urine.

One other issue of debate is the size of the squirt vs the size of the exit. The urethra is a visible opening. When we see the video, we see this huge stream of fluid.

The paraurethra ducts, or Skene's Glands, however, are a pair of TINY little holes. TINY!! They are virtually impossible to see they are so small. When I see a woman ejaculate an impressive volume, it just doesn't seem possible such a spray can come from such tiny little holes. But observing the urethra up close when it happens, I have SEEN that it isn't coming from there.

In videos, the way to tell the difference is to look at the volume coming out. If it's a single, solid stream, it's likely the water loading trick I mentioned. Ejaculation is more of a spray that just goes everywhere. In person, it's difficult to feel it on your hand which one it is. On your face though, should you be "australian kissing" when it happens, pee will hit you straight on the nose; ejaculation will go everywhere and soak everything. Australian kissing, for those who don't know, is just like French kissing, but you're down under.

It is common to feel the need to pee just before ejaculating. That's your brain, not your bladder. Stimulating the urethral sponge - the muscle that keeps pee in - can trigger the brain's association with that stimulation to mean that there is fluid in the bladder that needs to come out. And since you're told to drink volumes of water all the time, it is possible there is always a little pee in there. So, your brain's not wrong.

But, the OTHER function of the urethral sponge is to gather all that fluid and ejaculate. The brain is less familiar with that one. The brain still isn't wrong. It just has to catch up and learn the difference between the two. Something that helps to teach the brain is to incorporate something that the brain already associates with orgasm. Something like clitoral stimulation. Or use a vibrator on your clitoris while your partner stimulates your g-spot. Clitoral stimulation will teach your brain that the sensation can ALSO be associated with sexual pleasure. Your brain is always trying to make 2+2=4. Let's provide the 4 and the brain will figure out the equation. Once you learn the difference, and get a little practice, the difference will be an easy one to identify. But now, your brain only knows one thing and is trying to identify it with the closest thing it knows from experience.

Also, if your ejaculate smells or tastes like urine, that indicates that you're not hydrated properly. Lay off the sodas and drink lots of water. A woman should drink 1/2 your body weight in ounces of pure water a day. So, if you weigh 120, you should drink 60 ounces of water per day. Sure, it's possible it smells or tastes like urine because there actually is a little urine in there. But if your urine can be smelled or tasted, it still means you're not drinking enough water. Water helps dilute other chemicals and toxins in the body. Those chemicals and toxins are what give urine and ejaculate its color, odor and taste. Ideally, even urine will be practically odorless and tasteless, and mostly clear, except for whatever it is flushing from the body. Water aids in flushing those toxins and chemicals out. If you ARE drinking plenty of water, and a little urine gets mixed in, no one will notice.

For a healthy urethra, I also suggest to drink 8 ounces of cranberry juice per day. No. Cranberry juice doesn't technically cure a bladder infection or UTI. That will help flush out the bladder and urinary tract of toxins and irritants that can present like an infection. It will improve overall female health, and we all know that a healthy vagina works better. Drink pineapple juice to make the taste and smell sweet. A diet high in fruit will help in general too.

Empty your bladder completely before you play. That way, even when you feel the sensation to pee, you know that probably isn't it.

Put lots of puppy pads down (or towels, or whatever) and let it fly. If it's pee, so what. It's easily cleaned up. The only way you'll get past this is to let it fly and see what happens. I love the puppy pads. They're inexpensive. They absorb A LOT. And when play is done, you can throw them away. They even make earth friendly puppy pads now that will break down in the landfill. And nicest of all, you can have them around your house and no one will question it. That is, unless you don't have a dog. Maybe you should adopt a dog.

They also make GREAT ice breakers for the conversation where you have to tell a new boyfriend about your squirting ability. Not every man loves squirting as much as some others. Those guys would not be a good match for you. Better to find out over dinner than after you've drenched him and he's pissed off (no pun intended). Sit him down. Show him the puppy pads. And then say, "I have something I need to tell you." If he freaks and runs or makes a sour face, you're only out the cost of the puppy pads and didn't have to get naked to find out he isn't into it. Hopefully, he'll smile and say, "Cool!! Let's go!!"

You can also change how you view urine. Many women have deep issues about making a mess, peeing anywhere you're not supposed to, letting a partner touch your pee, etc. The result, while your brain is telling you that you need to pee, it is also feeding your guilt and shame. Next time you actually have to pee, touch the stream. See that it's fine. Wash your hands after. Get comfortable with it. Then do the same with your partner. This is not about golden showers, or water sports. This is about developing some comfort with a biological process that is interfering with a mental process. Your brain has to be comfortable to be able to ejaculate at first. If fear of it being urine is in the way, this is how you can overcome that.

All of that said, if someone is squeamish over a little pee, they should stick to masturbating. Alone. In the shower. Pee happens sometimes. Get over it. :)

Some notes on the smell and taste

Here are some generalities about the taste and odor. Even though these are usually true, one person's individual taste can be influenced by a variety of factors. Mostly, how everything combines inside the body. Figure in everything you eat and drink, add any medications you take and how much exercise you get and you get a unique flavor that is all yours. Part of your own unique pheromone system.

Diet has the most effect on any taste or odor. If a woman eats a balanced diet, with plenty of fruit and lots of plain ol' water, her taste will be very neutral and mostly flavorless. Fruits like pineapple, oranges (or tangerines) and strawberries can make it a little sweeter. Apples can make it very acidic and bitter, though. Green, stalk vegetables can make it quite unpleasant (asparagus, brussel sprouts for example). Too much red meat can also give it an unpleasant taste. Alcohol can effect the taste.

This is also true of a man's ejaculate.

For a woman, it can also be effected by her natural PH levels. At different times during her cycle, the taste or odor can be quite strong - even unpleasant sometimes, and there isn't enough pineapple juice in the world to correct it. Her natural musk, or pheromones, is stronger at times. That's just her natural scent. Embrace it!!

It is also my experience that different women all taste different at different times. Some, the smell and taste is stronger before her period or after. Some, before or after ovulation. Some, at the beginning or end of a play session. It seems as unique and individual as the woman. A CONSISTENT healthy diet with lots of fruit and water will help balance any fluctuation. But again, each woman is going to be a unique flavor to be enjoyed.

Overall health and any medications taken can effect the taste. ANY health condition or medication CAN have some effect, depending on the condition, medication and how the woman's health is effected generally by the condition or medication. This is another one the effect can be as unique as the woman. Diabetes generally makes the taste stronger, for example. Many cancer treatments can make the taste stronger. Many drugs taken for birth control or HRT seem to neutralize the taste somewhat. And in a bit of irony, the same drugs that rob the sex drive, can also neutralize the taste.

Last, exercise can effect the taste. Exercise makes things flow smoothly through the body and makes EVERYTHING in the body perform its best. Especially cardio. A lack of exercise can slow everything down to a crawl. The slower things flow through the body, the more likely they are to pick up toxins and contaminants from the body. Plenty of water and plenty of cardio can keep the taste neutral, which is the goal.

Question: "My girlfriend smokes and I can't stand the way her squirt smells and tastes."

Answer: Getting the smell or taste of nicotine in your mouth from female ejaculation is very unlikely. The offensive smell and taste from smoking is from the BURNING of the chemicals that are in commercial tobacco products. I'm not saying that nicotine isn't in her system and it isn't coming out when she squirts. I'm saying that nicotine, and even the other carcinogens in smoking, are quite odorless and tasteless by themselves. Except when burned. That's why they are so effective as pesticides. Even bugs can't smell it. The smell or taste you probably experienced was from poor diet and hydration and the way her body processes various toxins in her system. Less water concentrates other chemicals in the body and effects their smell and taste greatly. That's why sweat can smell toxic. Even tears will develop a strong odor from the chemicals in the body without enough water. They're all mucus based (mostly/kinda/sorta) and chemicals and toxins migrate into the mucus as the body's way of trying to rid you of those things.

Medication can also grossly effect the smell and taste. "Smells like pee; looks like pee, must be pee." Not necessarily. Some medications can effect the smell of your urine greatly. Actually, it is effecting the smell of ALL bodily fluids. But the brain makes a connection to urine and automatically labels that smell as urine, even if it isn't. Same with many other bodily odors. Again with the sweat. We "sweat" even when we're not noticeably/visibly perspiring. If we drink plenty of water, that sweat will be virtually odorless - even possibly attractive in the same way pheromones work with other animals.

"Baby, you're pretty."

"No. I just drink enough water and eat lots of strawberries."

If we don't, the smell can effect others' subconscious heavily.

"Dude! You need a shower!"

"No. Earlier I ate a big batter fried steak with some garlic marinated brussel sprouts and washed it down with a can of Red Bull and 3 Cokes."

The smell of cigarette smoke can be on her clothes and on her skin. It CAN leech out through the pores. If she's a heavy smoker, that is a more likely cause of the smell and taste. A thorough shower before playing should help. No, not saying she has a hygiene problem. I'm just proposing possible causes for the smell and taste that was asked about.

An ex used to eat onions on everything. "Onions are healthy," she would defend. And she's right. They are. And avocados. VERY healthy. She ate a bunch of those too. I did my best. But, I couldn't go down on her. Needless to say, we didn't date all that long.

Drink lots of water. LOTS. Eat lots of berries, pineapple and bananas because they make everything smell and taste better. Avoid foods that start with the letter "A" (Apples, avocados, asparagus for example) because they make everything smell and taste much worse. Get lots of cardio to help the body metabolize and cycle the crap out of the system.

Go Big Or Go Home

Those water cannon type squirting episodes are all about muscle control. Some activities strengthen the muscles that eject the fluid from the body. A wide variety of things. As the muscles surrounding the urethral sponge convulse and contract, it is possible to learn to shoot the ejaculate more forcefully. Proceed gently with "pushing" it out. Overworking those muscles can cause irritation in the urethra, which means it'll burn to pee. Not to confuse ejaculation with urination. Still two separate functions. But, the muscles for both are the same. Overexertion will have consequences.

Ejaculation and squirting are the same thing!! Just a difference in terminology. Even when the ejaculation doesn't literally shoot across the room like in porn, it is still ejaculation. Just like when men ejaculate, sometimes it squirts, sometimes it flows.

An ex, who I mentioned in a previous story, could hit the 8 ft. ceiling from the piledriver position on the bed. And, it was common for her to hit the wall about head high 10 ft away. All squirt, baby. In a single session (about an hour) on my kitchen floor, we managed to mop up a couple gallons of squirt. Another session, in the bathtub, with her standing against the back wall, she managed to fill the tub about 1/2" deep. I'm not sure if every woman is capable of delivering such monumental results. I imagine it depends on how hydrated a woman is and particularly how her body processes that water. I imagine that a fair amount of exercise will help keep the water flowing as it should. And I am guessing that a low sodium diet probably helped her body process the water best. That's just my theory and I concede it is possibly no more accurate than any other theory.

I will also share another anecdote on the legendary spraying of squirt. My goddaughter, I personally educated her on all things sexual. BTW, that is nowhere nearly as creepy and incestuous as it sounds. LOL. Think classroom, not bedroom.

Anyway. After she started college, she asked me about the g-spot. I drew her a diagram and sent her to her room, where she apparently found it. I explained to her about squirting and she apparently learned how. She then taught her girlfriend all about it. Ever since, one of the romantic things they do as a couple is have "squirt fights" in the kitchen when they are home alone (or at least THINK they're home alone). I have walked into the kitchen at their house more than once and almost busted my ass because it was still all over the floor. FYI. Lots and lots of squirt from two college girls on a tile floor is VERY slippery. Tread carefully. I also discovered it is quite slippery on the hardwood floor in the dining room after they had a squirt fight UNDER the table while they sat there having breakfast. It is also quite slippery on the cement floor in the garage, the wood on the patio, and most surprisingly, on the grass in the back yard.

Water Cannons

The "water canon" effect is not impossible. In fact, it's very easy to work up to. To help you get there, I have several recommendations.

1) Water. LOTS of water. The more you drink, the more you can squirt. You SHOULD be drinking 1/2 oz of water for every lb of body weight per day. If you weigh 100 lbs (for example), that's 50 ounces of water daily. That's for good health, not just for ejaculation prowess. But, you have to be careful to empty your bladder completely before you play.

2) KEGELS!!!!! I cannot recommend Kegels enough. One simple exercise that can improve overall vaginal health in a million ways. It will strengthen the muscles of your vagina like lifting weights. Just doing Kegels alone will increase your squirting pressure. Not only that, but Kegels will make the vagina more sensitive and improve the process of orgasm. Improving that process might give the squirting more intensity, and thus, more geyser-like effect.

3) Monitor your body. As an experienced squirter, you should be aware of the sensations you are experiencing as the ejaculation builds. Improve your awareness of those sensations. Keenly focus and learn every tiny detail of the process for YOUR body. Not just what the stimulation feels like, but everything. What it feels like when the fluid starts to build up all the way through what it feels like when it comes out. Everything.

4) Clean out thoroughly before you play, just like you would for anal play.

5) PUSH LIKE HELL!! If you've ever given birth, think of it kinda like that. At the moment when it starts to gush, PUSH! PUSH! PUSH! And keep pushing through the entire ejaculation. Timing is kinda important. You want to time the push for the precise moment that it begins and continue until you're done.

These steps should result in a significant improvement in your water canon effect. BUT, the pushing will possibly cause a little burning when you urinate (the first few times) because you will be straining the urethra slightly when you push. This will pass with experience. Ejaculation doesn't exit through the urethra, but pushing can strain it a little because it's the same muscle.

The more Kegels you do, the more this process will give you results. Kegels are the healthiest thing you can do for your vagina. It's possible they even prevent cancer and a wide range of medical conditions. Lots of Kegels can even alleviate menstrual cramps.

I have another article on this titled Pussy Yoga & The Cure For Cramps

And, since you are pushing hard, the cleaning out is VERY important to avoid a mess. Also, when you push hard like this, you MIGHT prolapse a little, vaginally or anally. Nothing to be concerned about (unless your anus stays prolapsed and it becomes painful). It should retreat as soon as you stop pushing. If it doesn't, you or your partner should be able to gently push it back in without a problem.

Also keep in mind that the Skeen's Glands (paraurethral openings) are tiny little holes. Your expectations of the volume of what comes out needs to be realistic. With practice, you can increase that volume dramatically. Unbelievably even. I've met several women that could shoot it like a fire hose with ease, and have talked to several others. I have also talked with some adult performers who can shoot an impressive stream. The suggestions above should help you build up to it.

Fisting

I talk a big game about fisting. I personally think it might be the most intimate thing a couple can do. The trust, intimacy and communication involved is totally next level. I bring it up with all this talk about squirting s because the most intense squirting I know of is with a hand inside. Seriously. Speaking in tongues and out of body experiences type intensity.

My favorite move is to roll my knuckles across her g-spot. Once they return to earth, women tell me it's nice. (grins)

If you want to experience it - and you DO want to experience it because most women say it is life-changing - you have to first believe it will fit. It isn't that it won't fit. For almost all women, it will. Maybe not the first time you try. Maybe not the 10th time. But, it WILL fit. Patience and lots of lube will get you there. You have to relax and surrender.

He also has to believe it will fit. But not be so cocky about it that he gets impatient. Just like with squirting, pressure is counter productive. He needs to be willing to learn the construction of your vagina. Regardless if he has fisted someone else, you are unique and he needs to recognize that. He needs to feel where your vagina gives and where it doesn't. Where your hip bones are. He needs to "warm things up" with some oral, which might have you tensed up again. Start slow and gentle. Baby steps and go from there.

When I was learning about fisting at Valentine's Fisting School, there was a lesbian woman who was only 19. She had never had a cock inside her, not even once. The most she'd ever had was a couple of WOMEN'S fingers. No children.

Her Domme dropped her in my lap for me to practice on. When I first started, her pussy was so tight that it cut the circulation off when I only had three fingers inside her. Valentine promised me it would work if I took my time. Her Domme told her to stay with me until the job was done. So, we worked on it for an hour. Took a break. Had some lunch and tried again for about an hour. I got four fingers in and she was fine. But from two hours of trying, she was getting VERY tender. So, we stopped and went to a movie. We had coffee after. We sat at the coffee shop for a couple hours and laughed about life. Then, we came back and tried again. Ten minutes later, I was in. Changed her life.

Yes. My hands are rather large. No problem. The problem IS NOT that your vagina is so tight. Remember, it's designed to pass an eight pound bowling ball. The problem is 1) YOU thinking it won't fit. 2) Patience of the person trying to fist you. 3) Experience. Experience tells me to believe and be patient. And, if it doesn't work the first time, take a break. Try again another time. Consistent practice is also important.

Stretching

Question: Various questions and conversations about fisting, stretching the vagina for bigger cocks and/or toys and pain during insertion of large cocks, toys, fists, etc..

Answer: Actually, Kegel exercises WILL help. The exercises strengthen the PC muscles. But, they also improve elasticity and circulation of the vaginal tissue. That means, they give your vagina some "range".

Anatomically speaking, naturally, the vagina has a range of expansion that is surprisingly wide. It's designed to allow a baby to exit. With plenty of lube, natural or not, sex should never be uncomfortable or painful. If it is, there may be a medical issue that needs to be addressed.

However, anxiety also has a wide range. It doesn't necessarily have to be a horrific, traumatic event to cause a sexual issue. It could be as simple as nervousness with the person you're having sex with. Or trust issues, or control issues or any one of a thousand VERY MINOR fears, possibly in some kind of combination with each other. All of which usually have a very simple and easy solution by identifying those things that make you nervous. I think often those anxieties are the result of rushing things. Just my opinion. Slow down and give things time.

Sex is the one place where all our masks come off. Whatever fears and anxieties a person has, they cannot hide them when they are naked and alone with the person they're getting freaky with. Most of those weird dysfunctions we all talk about are the result of some kind of VERY MINOR mindfuck that's going on in our heads that has been allowed to escalate into creating a behavioral or physiological result. For men, ED is often that physiological result; for women, it's often a pussy that says "NO" for some reason. Look for what causes the nervousness, find the cure for the undesired physiological reaction.

Related Question: "Will fisting (or large insertions of some kind) make it easier or harder to squirt?"

Answer: Both. Some women, it sends them over the edge and they squirt buckets when they are stretched open or filled so completely. For other women, the stretching seems to prevent them from being able to completely get over the finish line. They can orgasm wonderfully. But squirting seems to be impaired or blocked and whatever is inside them has to come out.

In the same genre, many women have difficulty squirting while a toy or penis is inside them. Pull the toy or penis out and they squirt normally. But inside, they just can't get there. For some women, this may be physical. There is something about the same stimulation that got them TO the edge, does not get them OVER the edge. Nothing wrong with that. Just a matter of learning what works and carrying on.

For others, it seems to be more of a mental block. They might still be holding on to the idea that it's pee or that they don't want to drench their partner, or something like that. For them, I (and their partners) can only remind them that it's safe to completely let go - not with words, but by being a man that is consistently safe and trustworthy. Hopefully, in time, they will.

Some of these women are holding back due to trust and safety issues. Not just when something is inside them, but any time they are on the edge of squirting. It could be that a previous partner didn't like them squirting and traumatized them for it. It could be all internal with them. Something in their brain is a hurdle they can't quite get over. In that case, only being a trustworthy, safe partner consistently is about all that can be done. Eventually, probably, something will click and she'll feel safe enough to let go. Until then, be patient and don't push.

Bottom line... There's still a lot to learn about topic. I have been fortunate to have plenty of partners to learn with, plenty of sources to learn from, and the opportunities to learn on my own. This is like everything else when it comes to sex. You don't have to know anything to have fun and as long as you approach everything with a childlike curiosity, you'll learn and you will continue to have lots of fun. Squirting is something where the grownups are ENCOURAGED to make a mess. How much fun is that, right?